Made in the USA
Monee, IL
24 October 2022

16464925R00070